How to Pass
NURSING EXAMS

Study Skills and Test-Taking Techniques

Sally Lagerquist, R.N., M.S.

Review Press

Acknowledgments

This book is a reality due to Jan Corcoran's creative influence, ongoing encouragement, and positive thinking; to Tom Lagerquist's sense of humor and perspective; and to Annette Cook's skill in managing my time as well as her infectious enthusiasm for detail and organization.

We also wish to thank Phoebe Helm for her ideas during the early developmental phase of this book.

Production Coordination: Matrix Productions
Copy-editing: Elliot Simon
Design: Merrill Peterson & Suzanne Marvier
Typesetting: Harrington-Young

To our daughter, Elana
and
Our son, Kalen
You have our gift of roots and wings
Enjoy developing your own blueprint for success

Contents

A Message to Nursing Students

Have you ever said to yourself: "No matter how hard I study, I don't do well on tests," or, "I know the material but my grades don't show it"? If so, this book is for you. In seven concise and practical chapters it presents such topics as: how to organize your time and study; how to memorize; how to increase your concentration; how to relax and control your test-related anxiety; and, finally, how to approach various examinations. Can test preparation and performance be improved? Most definitely, yes! How? By knowing how to learn the subject and by knowing how to take a test.

WHY I WROTE THIS BOOK

As a nurse educator with a special interest in improving study skills and test-taking abilities, I have come in contact over the last 25 years with many students who have shared a variety of problems associated with doing well in nursing school and on nursing exams. Their concerns range from anxiety about doing well on a test to a fear that their mind will go blank during an exam. Frustration about what to study, how to study, time management, how to organize, concentration difficulties, and poor recall are other concerns confronting students.

My background includes teaching at the School of Nursing, University of California at San Francisco, for over twelve years, at both the undergraduate and graduate levels, as well as in the Continuing Education Department, where I met many nurses from other parts of the country as well as Canada, Europe, Asia, and Africa. These experiences provided me with invaluable opportunities to learn about the academic problems students face at various phases in their nursing education; in turn, I have developed and tested approaches on how to help nursing students make learning easier for themselves and how to do better in nursing school. After teaching these skills for the past ten years, I have been asked repeatedly by those who attended my courses to put my ideas and practical suggestions in writing.

WHAT MAKES THIS BOOK DIFFERENT

You can use this book throughout nursing school as well as in prenursing courses and even after you have graduated, because the ideas and approaches presented are practical, a result of applied common sense and proven success with many types of students. Some topics (for example, *how to take efficient lecture notes*, and *how to master the text book*) are more important at the beginning of nursing school; other topics might become significant later (for example, *how to increase concentration, and how to improve your memory*). These ideas are not limited to one nursing subject or a single year in nursing school. The principles apply to almost any situation.

These study skills can be mastered quickly. The step-by-step methods will help you develop organizational skills essential to your academic success. The chapters are short enough to read within a brief period of time. This means you will be able to apply these skills directly to your assignments *right now;* you will be better able—in your current courses—

to establish priorities, organize and remember the material, and take tests with better results. You can read the chapters in any order that meets your immediate needs. Skip, skim, or select any topic—this will make for productive, enjoyable use of your time.

THE PURPOSE OF THIS BOOK

This book is designed as a guide to greater success in nursing school. You will find suggested techniques to help you efficiently and effectively use your study/learning/review time to take useful notes, to master the material in as short a time as possible, and to see better results on exams (and have more time for other aspects of life and living in addition to school!).

In short, this book is designed to help you learn how to learn. May it bring you good results in nursing school and on your exams. Enjoy reading it!

Sally Lagerquist

1

Introduction

WHY IS TEST-TAKING A "NEGATIVE" EXPERIENCE?

The test-taking situation is viewed as negative because often there is no other way to gain the reward of entry into nursing practice. Something important is riding on one's test performance—the RN license. For some people—that is, nurses reentering practice who need to take courses for continuing education or licensure renewal—test-taking is a negative experience because they do not know the material or do not know how to take tests or have become anxious because they have been away from tests so long. Those who are slow readers may worry about not having enough time to finish the exam or not comprehending the exam language. Thus, two people having a similar level of knowledge can get widely different scores on the same test because one person has better test-taking skills or more experience in taking tests or is less anxious.

TEST WISENESS

Being "test-wise" does not mean beating the test, for one's score is not a matter of chance or lucking-out. It is not a matter of deciphering a code or figuring out the gimmicks. It is not a system for second-guessing the test writer. Neither is test-wiseness a substitute for knowledge, for you do need knowledge. With a well-constructed test, being test-wise will not enable someone with inadequate knowledge to score high.

Someone who is test-wise is not born that way. Test-wiseness involves a set of skills that can be improved through practice and instruction. And having acquired the skills does not mean that you will therefore always score high. But by increasing your test-taking proficiency, you can decrease the associated anxiety and thereby raise your test scores.

What then is test-wiseness? It is the ability to utilize relevant cues in the test or test situation to obtain a score consistent with your level of proficiency. Test-wiseness should be used as an approach to the test situation. It is *not* a substitute for knowledge. Even when you can pick up the cues to correct options, knowledge of the subject matter is usually required to fully utilize those cues. But knowing how to take tests *can* help you to overcome inadequate test-taking abilities, demonstrate what you know to the fullest degree possible in a test situation, and improve your chance of success on exams.

HOW TO DO YOUR BEST ON A TEST

The most important thing you need to achieve peak perform-ance on a test is a goal. A goal keeps you on target and helps you self-correct your weak points. You need a goal that is concrete: passing NCLEX-RN. You need a goal that is realis-tic: getting about 70% of the 372 questions on the NCLEX-RN exam correct to pass. And you need to make the goal your *own* goal, not your school's goal. Your goal for the NCLEX should be to pass, not to score at Phi Beta Kappa level. You also need to set priorities among your goals. For example, today the exam is my priority; tomorrow, life! You need to picture your goal, to picture yourself taking the exam and passing it. And you need to imprint this image and follow through in the real world.

You need to let your goal happen. How? By

    a. Learning relaxation techniques.
    b. Learning concentration exercises.
    c. Rehearsing mentally.

Learn at the level at which you perform best. Learn self-talk. Learn phrases of affirmation. And then mentally execute the self-talk. "Soon it will all be over"; "I will take one problem at a time."

There are two roads to failure: (1) a lack of involvement in what you are doing, that is, a lack of seriousness; and (2) a lack of relentlessness, that is, not being a studyholic when that is most essential.

You need to establish personal goals as your strongest source of motivation. You need a high level of commitment. It is okay to be obsessed by the outcome, as long as that obsession is limited in time. Make your goal long-range, intermediate-range, or short-range. The goal should also be a challenging but realistic one. You must have a deep belief that you will reach your goal. The clearer you visualize the goal, the more you will kindle the desire to reach it and the more exhilarating that feels. Remember what all your efforts are aimed at: achieving passing scores so you can get your RN license.

2

Myths and Facts about Test-Taking

Myth	Fact
You need an inborn gift to be good at test-taking.	Test-taking skills can be learned.
You never do well on tests; therefore you'll never get any better.	Practice, knowledge of test-taking cues, effective and efficient ways of mastering content, taking notes, and test-wiseness *can* all improve your performance on tests.
Doing well on tests is a matter of luck.	Psychological studies show that a person's luck is largely influenced by his or her state of mind. Tests show, for example, that a negative or "beat" state of mind attracts bad luck; a negative attitude slows your reflexes and dulls your perceptions, causing you to misjudge situations and overlook key words. A University of Chicago study found that the mental attitude of students distinctly influenced their success in performing a task. A

Myth	Fact
	person expecting to do poorly will make errors or oversights that confirm her or his negative expectations, saying, in effect, "I didn't think I'd be able to do it. And you see, I'm right!" Psychiatrists at the University of Chicago have also found a marked tendency for unlucky things to happen to a person who is unhappy with herself or himself. Thus, luck is to a large extent self-generated. So if you want to change your luck, change your attitude.
If you are test-wise, you don't need knowledge.	The test-wise person does not have a mystical ability to get the right answer. That individual has learned to respond to cues within the test. However, this ability is directly proportional to the number of cues in the test. More often than not, the unanxious exam taker familiar with the subject matter will do better than someone who relies heavily on cues.
In order to pass, you must get all the answers correct.	There's no perfect score to attain. For NCLEX-RN you only need to *pass*; it is scored on a pass-or-fail basis.
When in doubt, it is always better to guess.	Find out first if there is a built-in penalty for guessing. If there is, do not guess. When in doubt about the penalty, it is better to leave the question alone, because, although nothing is gained in terms of points, neither are points deducted.
When in doubt, do not guess.	It might be wise to guess when you have narrowed down the four options to two. You need to say to

Myth	Fact
	yourself, "I *know* it is one of these two," rather than, "I do *not* know which of these two." "*If* I know it is one of these two, I will guess." This is called educated guessing.
You get partial credit for the next-best answer.	You get credit *only* for selecting the best answer.
You should spend most of your test time mastering the difficult questions.	First you should answer the easy questions. Do not waste time and energy, nor dissipate your confidence, by zeroing in on the most difficult ones first. They will drag you down, and you will run out of time and lose points on the easy ones.
It is usually helpful to go back and change answers.	Your first hunch usually is your best, unless as you proceed through the exam you uncover further information that disqualifies your first hunch.
When in doubt choose the answer that matches what you have seen performed by a physician.	The NCLEX test is for RNs; therefore the best answers (unless specifically designated in the case situation preceding the question) are those appropriate for the role and the scope of function of the RN, *not* the MD.

3

The Ultra-Successful Test-Taker

THE LOW SCORER VERSUS THE SUCCESSFUL TEST-TAKER

Low Scorer	Successful Test-Taker
• Loses track of time	• Is aware of time, knows time limits
• Spends excessive time on one question	• Budgets time
• Gives up on difficult or complex questions	• Attempts every question, breaking complex questions down into elements
• Proceeds without understanding directions	• Reads directions carefully
• Spends more time on certain questions (as if differential weight were given to certain questions, although in reality all questions may be weighted equally in terms of points).	• Knows how questions will be scored. Adjusts time accordingly; that is, will *not* spend more time on some items *if* all questions are weighted equally.
• Guesses wildly when there's a	• Does not guess wildly when

Low Scorer	*Successful Test-Taker*
penalty for guessing	points can be deducted for incorrect responses
• Misreads or misinterprets key words	• Is alert to key terms
• Passively stares at problems, hoping that correct answers will somehow materialize (in other words, uses wishful thinking)	• Actively reasons out the questions. Uses continuous, aggressive thinking to "attack" the problem
• Reads into a question something that was not intended by the test-writer	• Takes a question at face value. Anticipates what the answer is likely to be and then looks for it among the options. For instance, anticipates that the answer is likely to be a reason if the question asks "why"
• Jumps at the first likely option rather than suspending selection until all options have been read	• Considers all four options even though the first one seems the best
• Continues to hold on to an anticipated answer even though it isn't among the options. Tries to force the anticipated answer to fit	• Discards an anticipated answer when it is not among the options, and relates each option to the question
• Misreads directions: chooses a "correct" statement as the best answer when the question actually asks, "Which of the following is *not* appropriate."	• Identifies key words, eg. *not, except*
• Gets stuck on two options that are close	• Studies options that are similar and *compares* them with each other to see what makes them *different*
• Freezes; focuses continuously on *all* 4 options	• Uses a process of elimination to free up concentration on fewer options. For example, eliminates two options to be able to focus on the two remaining choices
• Selects an option that is not	• When two options look good,

Low Scorer	Successful Test-Taker
comprehensive enough	chooses the one that encompasses both options
• Chooses options that include exact, global terms, such as "always" or "none"	• Chooses options that use gray terms, such as "usually," "generally," "many," or "on the average"
• Doesn't use analysis or systematic procedure • Doesn't reason logically	• Systematically breaks the stem down into elements and uses logical reasoning, eg. read the following directions: **Cross out the letter after the letter in the word "seldom" which is in the same position in the word as it is in the alphabet.**
• Does not break a question down into manageable units and proceed systematically	A successful test taker would start by reading the first step: *"cross out the letter...*, then say: "I have to find a letter to cross out ... *'after the letter'."* The person would then say, "First I have to find another letter in the word." Then, reading, "First find the word *'seldom'"* The successful test-taker says, "That's the word; now what letter in the word 'seldom' is in the *same position in the word...as it is in the alphabet?*
• Has a "know, don't-know" attitude. If the answer doesn't come to mind right away, feels lost • Reasons through partway, and then gives up if the solution is not obvious. Gives up too soon if it's too hard, if it doesn't make sense, or if it's too complicated • Relies strictly on hunches, not logical reasoning and systematic	The successful test-taker says, "I know D is the fourth letter in the alphabet and the fourth letter in 'seldom'...but wait, I must *'cross out the letter after that.'* That means don't cross out D, but O (seldøm)." • Analyzes and sees relationships

Low Scorer	*Successful Test-Taker*
analysis of the options in the stem	
• Seldom rereads or goes back over the test	• Uses extra time to go over key words
• Spends more time rereading alternatives	• Analyzes the stem carefully
• Rushes through or skips directions	• For example, Person A says, "I taught my dog to whistle." Person B says, "Funny, I never heard him whistle." Person A says, "I *taught* him, I didn't say he *learned* it."
• Tries to remember solutions to similar problems rather than solve each new problem independently	• Avoids preset solutions
• Uses a negative approach; that is, chooses an answer only because the others are not good	• Chooses the *best* answer, one that seems *good* or *better* than others
• Chooses words that are unfamiliar	• Avoids unfamiliar options

ATTITUDES SUPPORTING PEAK PERFORMANCE ON TESTS

The successful test-taker says:

"It's okay to say this exam is not the most important thing in my life."

"I can finish."

"It's okay to not answer all the questions."

"This too shall pass. The exam is but an incident, an episode, not the major event in my life."

"I deserve a reward" (and plans a reward after the test is over).

The successful test-taker also laughs instead of cries, by putting things in perspective with a sense of humor.

ANALYZE YOUR OWN TEST-TAKING ERROR PATTERNS

Most of the errors students make in taking tests fall into patterns. This is primarily because such errors are learned. And the more you repeat them, the harder they are to change. However, once you have recognized that the errors are learned, that they have a pattern and are not just random, you can focus on strategies to remedy them and remove them from your test-taking behavior. This is very similar to those who feel they are poor spellers. If you stop and analyze your spelling errors, they will usually fall into two or three categories—words you do not know, and more common words that you have learned incorrectly.

Listed below you will find *fifteen categories* of test-taking errors, derived from my ten years of assisting thousands of nursing students throughout the country to improve their test-taking skills. As you study these categories you will discover that they are not mutually exclusive; that is, your error may fit in more than one category. When this happens, place the item in the category you believe best explains the reason for your error, or place it in all of the categories to which it applies until you are able to narrow down your own error pattern. As you study these categories you will also note that I did not include such statements as "I read too much into the item." Even though students often do that and faculty often tell students that, I have not found it useful as a category because it does not assist you to focus specifically enough on an error to remedy it.

To acquaint yourself with the fifteen categories, first read through them and think about them. Second, answer the thirteen questions that follow the category list and analyze your answers. Don't worry about the number you miss at this point. Once you have decided which category or categories your error belongs in, place the number of that item to the left of the category or categories that you think best explains your error. After you have completed the thirteen items and checked your answers and categorized them, compare your categories with the categories and explanations that follow the questions. Remember, the important thing at this point is to become familiar with the process, not how many you get right.

Categorization of Test-Taking Errors

1. I chose an example rather than a concept or vice versa. (This also applies to answers that are too narrow as compared to a more inclusive answer.)
2. I chose an answer I did not understand because the answer I knew seemed too simple.
3. I chose a "good" answer, but it was not the most immediate priority.
4. I failed to note an important word or phrase in the stem, such as "all but," "except," "not," "always," "first," "most important," "most immediate."
5. I focused on the medical need and ignored the psychological need.
6. I chose the wrong answer because I did not know the information.
7. I failed to keep in mind the patient's age when I answered the question.
8. I chose an answer that was too judgmental or did not elicit the patient's involvement.
9. I chose an answer that failed to seek additional information.
10. I chose an answer that was too definitive or inflexible.
11. I allowed an unfamiliar technical word (or one I was unsure of) to throw me off the track, and I failed to utilize the rest of the information in the item.

12. I chose an answer that did not fit the criticalness of the situation.
13. I chose an answer that was very similar to another alternative without realizing that if one were correct the other would also be correct. (For example, if rapid were correct, then fast would also be correct when talking about speed.)
14. I avoided choosing an answer I knew to be right because I thought that alternative might not be available in a real-life situation.
15. Other (*Note:* Before placing an item in this category first see if it fits one of the other categories. At the end, see if you can determine a pattern for the errors you've put in this category.)

Sample Questions (Items)

1. When a patient asks you why he can't take insulin by mouth, explain that insulin taken by mouth is destroyed by:
   A. Digestive enzymes.
   B. Hydrochloric acid.
   C. Glucagon hydrochloride.
   D. Polypeptide chains.

2. Which of the following statements about breastfeeding is true?
   A. Breastfeeding is always safer and more satisfying for the baby than is formula-feeding.
   B. Breastfeeding can be a distasteful experience to some mothers even though they really do love their babies.
   C. Breastfeeding cannot be a satisfying experience for mother or baby unless a mother really wants to feed the baby in this fashion.
   D. Statements B and C only.
   E. None of the above.

3. If a pregnant woman expresses indecision about whether or not to breastfeed, which of the following

replies would be most appropriate for the nurse to make?

A. "Your baby will feel more loved and more secure if you breastfeed him."

B. "Maybe you won't have enough milk to breast-feed anyhow. Why don't you wait until after he is born and decide then on the basis of the milk available."

C. "There certainly are advantages and disadvantages to all methods of feeding. What have you considered so far in trying to decide on a method?"

D. "Breast milk is the best possible food for a baby, and if you are willing to sacrifice your figure, you certainly should give the baby this advantage."

4. How can an expectant father be most helpful to his wife during pregnancy?

A. By supervising her diet and activities to make sure she follows instructions.

B. By accepting the fact that her attention has been temporarily withdrawn from him and become centered on herself and the child.

C. By protecting her from all responsibility and problems during her pregnancy.

D. By helping her keep busy so she won't become too introspective.

5. Anxiety and fear in a pregnant woman may cause:

A. Failure to assimilate an adequate diet.

B. Overeating and excessive weight gain.

C. A higher incidence of labor complications.

D. Hyperactivity of the fetus.

E. All of the above.

6. The Moro reflex is a response to:

A. Disturbance of orientation in space.

B. Falling sensation.

C. Loud noises.

D. Any of the above.

7. If a nurse observes an infant gagging on mucus and

becoming cyanotic, the nurse should first:
A. Call the doctor.
B. Aspirate the pharynx with a catheter.
C. Raise the baby's head and slap it on the back.
D. Give oxygen by positive pressure.

8. In order to understand the preadolescent boy, parents need to accept the fact that:
   A. Friends in his peer group are extremely important to him.
   B. He moves between dependence and independence.
   C. He is likely to withdraw when frustrated.
   D. He rejects his parents because he does not want to feel dependent on them.

9. Which of the following nurses will probably have the most "discipline problems" with a group of hospitalized adolescent boys?
   A. Miss A, who will not tolerate swearing or bad language.
   B. 19-year-old Miss B, who tells them exactly what she expects.
   C. Miss C, who plays the guitar.
   D. Miss D, who never argues with them.

10. Which of the following statements about rooming-in is *not* true?
    A. Rooming-in is a development of the 20th century.
    B. Rooming-in reflects the attitude that care should be attuned to the needs of the family as a unit with interacting members.
    C. Rooming-in provides parents opportunities to learn about the care of the new baby in an atmosphere where help is always available.
    D. Rooming-in requires special preparation of hospital staff.

11. Which of the following plans would probably be least effective in helping a parent deal with sibling rivalry?

A. Realistically including children in planning family activities.
B. Scheduling parents' time so that each child receives an equal share of time.
C. Making a point of listening to each child's questions and stories.
D. Recognizing the unique attributes and problems of each child.

Six-year-old June Farrelly is brought to the emergency room by her mother. Half an hour ago she was bitten on her right arm by a neighbor's dog.

12. The recommended first step in emergency treatment of a child with a dog bite is to:
   A. Thoroughly cleanse the area with soap and water.
   B. Report the accident to the police.
   C. Encourage free bleeding.
   D. Cauterize the wound and suture it.

13. June should receive active immunization unless:
   A. The dog cannot be found.
   B. Evidence of central nervous system disorder occurs.
   C. There is evidence that the dog was rabid.
   D. The wound seems superficial.

Answers:

1. A; 2. B; 3. C; 4. B; 5. E; 6. D; 7. B; 8. B; 9. B; 10. A; 11. B; 12. A; 13. B.

Categorization and Explanation of Answers

1. If you missed item one, that was probably for one of three reasons (error categories 1, 2 or 11):
   1. You may not have recognized *digestive enzymes* as the most inclusive answer, OR

2. You may have fallen for one of the more difficult (technical) terms.
3. A combination of error categories 2 and 11. Decide if you missed it because A seemed too simple or because you were unsure of the terms used in B, C, and D.

2. If you missed item two, check error categories 4, 8, and 10 to see if:
   1. You failed to notice the word *true*, or *always*, OR
   2. You chose an answer which was too judgmental or inflexible.

3. If you missed item three, check error categories 8 and 9 to see if:
   1. You were too judgmental or failed to elicit the patient's involvement, OR
   2. You did not seek additional information—in this case, what the patient was considering, which would have told you about her feelings and her knowledge.

4. If you missed item four, check error categories 5, 8, and 10 to see if:
   1. You focused on her physical needs and ignored who should have responsibility for meeting those needs or ignored her psychological need to be accepted while she focused more on herself and the baby (temporarily) than on her husband, OR
   2. You chose an answer that was too judgmental or too definite. (Notice the terms *supervise, protect,* and *too introspective;* they are too definite, implying that she is a child, whereas the word *accept* is much more appropriate to her psychological needs.

5. If you missed item five, you probably ignored the phrase *may cause* in the stem (check error category 4). *May cause* merely indicates a possibility, not that it has to or must cause any of the problems listed.

6. If you missed item six, check error category 11. You may have forgotten what *Moro* means; however, if you had focused on the term *reflex* (which you *do* know), you would have recognized that A, B, and C are all reflexes and that A is just a restatement of B. Thus, you could have gotten the correct answer, D, just by utilizing your knowledge of reflexes as automatic responses.

7. If you missed item seven, check error categories 12 and 14 to see if:
   1. You failed to note the criticalness of the situation (the baby is turning blue), OR
   2. You hesitated choosing B because you know a catheter is not always available; however, its being mentioned in answer B means you should assume it was available. Did you refuse to use it when it was the best answer? Also note that in this case C and D would do more harm than good.

8. If you missed item eight, check error category 1. You have chosen an example (A, C, and D are true statements, though examples of a concept or underlying principle—B) rather than the broader concept, B, which explains why A, C, and D are true statements. When facing items of this sort, the more encompassing concept is almost *always* the best answer, since it represents a broader understanding on which to base your nursing behaviors.

9. First of all, with item nine, you should recognize that it is a poor item. However, from time to time you may encounter poor items. When this happens give the item very little time; just give it your best and most reasonable guess and go on; don't let it upset you. Now, let's see if you can do that with item nine. If you are dealing with a group of hospitalized adolescent boys, you recognize that there is a strong probability that they will be "getting the attention and approval of their peers." This is probably going to be even more so if the nurse (the authority figure in this case) is near their age. Since alternative B is

the only alternative which mention's the nurse's age and since this alternative also includes setting parameters, B would be the best answer (recognizing that this is a poor item). This item would fit error category 15 as well as category 7.

10. If you missed item 10, check error categories 4 and 13 to see if:
    1. You failed to notice the word "not" in the item.
    2. You forgot to reason through alternative A, recognizing that the term "rooming-in" may be new but the concept of newborns staying in the room with their families is old.
    3. You noticed that alternatives B, C, and D are all true statements.

11. If you missed item eleven, check error categories 1 and 4 to see if:
    1. You chose a concept rather than an example. For example, the *concept* underlying sibling rivalry is the need for each child to be recognized and treated as a unique individual. This *concept* is best stated in alternative D. Alternatives A, B, and C are *examples* of methods some parents might use in recognizing the uniqueness of each child.
    2. You might have read it as "most" rather than "least" in this item. While D represents the *concept*, B would represent the *least* effective alternative because the term "equal share" implies that parents should give each child the same amount of time regardless of his or her unique needs or attributes.

12. If you missed item twelve, check error categories 3 and 4 to see if:
    1. You failed to respond to the most immediate priority.
    2. You noticed the term "first step" in the item.

13. If you missed item thirteen, check error categories 4, 6, and 12 to see if:

1. You failed to notice the criticalness of the situation implied in alternative B. If "central nervous system disorder occurs," you would suspect that it is too late for "active immunization" (which, as you know, is a live virus, in this case rabies) to be of any value.
2. You did not know that rabies affects the central nervous system; thus, you did not realize that it would be too late to give an "active immunization."
3. You did not know that "active immunization" is a live virus designed to trigger the body's immune system to prepare to fight a particular virus which may invade the system. This is similar to the rationale for immunizing children against measles, mumps, and polio.
4. You failed to notice the term "unless" in item thirteen.

Summarizing the Errors You Made on the Thirteen Practice Items

To illustrate how to summarize the types of errors made in taking tests of this type, let's summarize the errors involved in the thirteen practice items you have just completed. For purposes of illustration, let's assume that you missed all of the items for all the reasons (error categories) I suggested. Then your summary would appear as on chart 1.

Now it is fairly easy to see that error category 4 was of influence in your missing six items. Thus this would be the most important category of errors to start eliminating from your test-taking behaviors. Error categories 1 and 8 were of influence in your missing three items each; thus, you would want to focus on eliminating these types of errors as well. Perhaps three categories of errors are enough to focus on eliminating at one time.

Please practice additional items, focusing on eliminating the errors represented by categories 1, 4 and 8. To do this

Chart 1

Error Category	Items Answered Incorrectly Due to the Influence of this Error Category
1.	1, 8, 11
2.	1
3.	12
4.	2, 5, 10, 11, 12, 13
5.	4
6.	13
7.	9
8.	2, 4, 3
9.	3
10.	2, 4
11.	1, 6
12.	7, 13
13.	10
14.	7
15.	9

choose 25–30 items from the *Q and A Practice Book.** Once you have completed these items, check the answers and analyze any errors you made. Your primary goal at this point is to have made fewer errors involving categories 1, 4 and 8. After meeting this goal, move on to other categories which you wish to eliminate. The format for each of your practice exercises should be: Complete 25–30 items in the *Q and A Practice Book*; then, check your answers and analyze your errors. From your summary, determine your progress toward your goal, set new goals and/or categories to work on and repeat the process.

Once you have eliminated your most frequent error categories from your test-taking behavior you may want to work on speed. The goal should be to complete one item per minute. To do this, choose 30 items from the *Q and A Practice Book*, set a timer for thirty minutes or set your watch at twelve o'clock and begin answering the items.

Practice Questions & Answers for NCLEX-RN. Review for Nurses Tapes, Inc., San Francisco, CA: 1989.

Ignore the time, concentrating only on completing the items, until you have finished the items or the timer goes off. If you find you cannot answer 30 items in 30 minutes, set your goal at 20 items in 30 minutes and gradually increase your goal for each practice set until you can complete 30 items in 30 minutes (or perhaps you'd rather continue until you can complete 30 items in 25 minutes).

As the date of your RN Licensure Examination approaches, you will want to practice test-taking in 1½-hour blocks, since that is the way the test is administered. To do this, choose 90 items, set your watch at 12 o'clock and begin. Continue this process until you are able to complete all of the items before 1:30. The advantage of setting your watch at 12 is that you make the calculation easier and faster. If you glance at your watch at 12:45, you should have completed 45 items. If you glance at your watch at 1:10 you should have completed 70 items and so on. Time is important on standardized tests, so hints such as this one can be helpful.

ANALYZE YOUR OWN TEST-TAKING SKILLS

In order to add to your test-taking techniques, you may need to analyze your skills further. The following may serve as an additional checklist. To use this chart, select and answer practice questions from any unit of *Addison-Wesley's Nursing Examination Review* by Sally Lagerquist. Look up the correct answers, then for each incorrect answer place a check mark next to the type of problem you had answering that question. Remember, there may be more than one reason for answering a particular question incorrectly. Look for which problems occur most frequently.

Repeat this procedure two more times, using different practice questions. This exercise should help you identify and reduce your test-taking problems.

Problem	*Practice 1*	*Practice 2*	*Practice 3*
1. Difficulty narrowing the four given options down to two			

Problem	Practice 1	Practice 2	Practice 3
2. Difficulty deciding between two best options and, instead, selecting the second-best answer			
3. Difficulty choosing the best option when all four options appear good			
4. Difficulty choosing the best option when none of them look good			
5. Looking for the right answer, which doesn't seem to be among the choices			
6. Not completing the test during the time allowed because too much time was spent on certain items (problem of budgeting time)			
7. Overthinking, reading beyond what is written in the stem			
8. Second-guessing an item's intent ("It *couldn't* be this simple.")			
9. Leaving too many answers blank			
10. Guessing wildly when scoring includes a correction for guessing			
11. Missing the meaning of key words and qualifying terms (for example, *first* action)			
12. Choosing responses with global terms (for example, "always," "none," "all," "never")			
13. Lack of basic knowledge (facts, theory, principles that are not learned or are learned incorrectly or vaguely)			

Problem	Practice 1	Practice 2	Practice 3
14. Selecting the option opposite in meaning to the actual best response			
15. Choosing an option that doesn't meet the condition of the stem (for example, stem asks for a *reason;* option selected is an *example*)			
16. Inaccurate reading of the directions in the stem			
17. Rereading the distractors many times instead of rereading the stem			
18. Selecting a *broad, general* response when the stem calls for *specific,* detailed response (or vice versa)			
19. Looking for an answer memorized from the textbook when the stem requires an "analysis" or "application of knowledge" type response			
20. Difficulty in selecting the best response when the stem has a negative term such as "not" or "except"			
21. Marking the wrong spot on the answer sheet			
22. Selecting an answer that is not understood and doesn't make sense to the examinee			
23. Selecting a response that is idealistic, controversial, or unrealistic rather than the typical, safe, or general response			
24. Selecting a response that is inappropriate to the intended scope and level of the exam			

Problem	Practice 1	Practice 2	Practice 3
(for example, choosing an answer appropriate to the role of the MD rather than the beginning practitioner RN)			
25. Choosing an option that is an example of or could be subsumed under a more comprehensive option			
26. Selecting a response that includes nontherapeutic communication. For example, denying a person's feelings, changing the subject, giving advice			
27. In questions on interpersonal relationships, choosing "there and then" responses rather than "here and now"; focusing on facts rather than feelings; focusing on fantasies rather than reality; focusing on interpreting behavior rather than supporting coping behavior			
28. Mathematical items (conversions, calculations, dosages, etc.)			

ENVIRONMENTAL DISTRACTIONS

It is important to identify and eliminate or minimize negative influences in your environment.

Internal Environment

Perfectionism may limit your success. The pressure of wanting to perform perfectly often impedes performance. If you feel you cannot afford to make a mistake, you take too much time deciding which option to choose. Another example of an internal distraction is *getting fixated* on an item. You take too much valuable time when you are unable to progress to other questions. Another internal distraction is *lacking awareness of time*. Don't let time get away from you, lose track of time, or make poor use of time when deciding which questions to answer first and how long to take.

External Environment

External distractions can also limit your success on tests. For example, your home environment may be one of discord. If you are fatigued or have been missing sleep, it will be difficult to concentrate or think clearly. If you are ill, you won't be able to perform at peak level. If you are worried about matters unrelated to the test, you may be unable to block out your anxieties during the test.

An external environment that is physically uncomfortable—for example, too cold or too hot—can impede your performance. However, an environment that is cold usually helps to keep you awake and alert. If the room is too hot or stuffy, or you're wearing heavy clothes, you may get drowsy, even semistuporous, and therefore not function well. Being on medications may cloud your senses, slow your reflex time and thinking time, and dull the clarity of your thought. Too much noise or too many people in the environment can serve as external distractions.

Finally, fear of loss of face about not doing well should be avoided. Many people enter an exam believing it would be a shame and embarrassment not to do well: "My brother did well, my mother did well, my family expects it of me; they have sacrificed time and money so that I could get someplace."

4
Learning the Material

TIME MANAGEMENT

Do the following symptoms of poor time management sound familiar to you?

- I never accomplish the things I plan to do.
- Look at my desk! It's cluttered with papers. I reshuffle them, but I never seem to clear them away.
- I frequently work overtime and spend more time doing things than I had originally planned.
- I'm continually being interrupted when I'm trying to study.
- I spend so much of my time on small, unimportant items that there's no time left for the important, complicated things that give me trouble.

If any of these statements seem familiar, you need to learn how to manage your time effectively. How you use your time depends on what you want to get done, so the first step is to establish goals. Because you are reading this book, we can assume that your primary goal at this time is to pass the RN licensure exam. Having established your goal, you need to develop a strategy for achieving it. Using time efficiently is an important element of that plan.

Since your habits play a part in how you manage time, you need to analyze how you currently spend your time. Make several copies of the blank form on page 29, and use it for a week to record how you spend each hour. Then, looking at the information you've collected, answer some questions:

- What are your most productive times of the day? your least productive?
- What activities could you eliminate or reduce to make time for study?
- How or where are you wasting time?

Use the answers to these questions and the guidelines below to make up a weekly schedule that includes adequate study time. Fill in that schedule on another copy of the blank form.

GUIDELINES FOR SCHEDULING STUDY TIME

The following guidelines will help you draw up a study schedule, whether for a single exam or a school quarter.

1.   *Decide how long to study.* Although one rule of thumb says you should study two hours for every hour in class, such an approach is not necessarily effective at all times. How long you need to study will vary from subject to subject. Let experience be your guide. Adjust your study time so that you can master the material, not simply read it. Then, when you've estimated how long it will take to master a study unit, double the figure! It's better to be realistic than to end up trying to write a 3,000-word paper the night before it's due or to memorize all the bones in the body in an hour!

2.   *Plan blocks of time.* Psychological research studies show that people use time most efficiently in one-hour blocks: 50 minutes of study, 10 minutes' break.

	AM 6:00	7	8	9	10	11	PM 12	1	2	3	4	5	6	7	8	9	10	11	12
Mon																			
Tues																			
Wed																			
Thurs																			
Fri																			
Sat																			
Sun																			

3.   *Try to plan study times for immediately after classes.* Reviewing your lecture notes immediately after class facilitates retention and comprehension.

4.   *Prioritize your study time.* Put your time where your problem is! Study the most important, most difficult things first so you won't run out of time or energy before you get to them.

5.   *Use daylight hours if possible.* Research shows that, for most people, each hour of daylight study is equal to 1½ hours of nighttime study. But you must take your own biological rhythms into account. Plan to study when you are at your most alert and productive. If you are a "night owl," plan to study at night—make study your top nighttime priority.

6.   *Schedule time to sleep and to eat regular, nourishing meals.* Low energy, irritability, and fuzzy thinking can result from lack of sleep and improper nourishment. Be nice to yourself.

7.   *Give yourself time for living.* Work smarter, not longer. Working more hours does not necessarily mean getting more done. Leisure is as necessary as sleep and food for peak performance.

8.   *Don't become a slave to your schedule.* Don't get so caught up in scheduling that you waste time that would be better spent studying.

9.   *Be flexible.* Make each unit of study time productive. If nothing is getting through despite your best efforts, stop. An hour of gardening, shopping, exercise, or reading might be more productive right then.

TAKING NOTES

It is a common difficulty when preparing for an exam to realize that you have not taken good lecture notes and, therefore, your study aids are limited. Perhaps your notes are too skimpy or too cryptic. But more likely they are voluminous; they look like another textbook, and nothing makes sense. To alleviate your note-taking problems, try the *5R* method: *record, reduce, recite, reflect,* and *review.*

1.   Record. Take an 8½ by 11-inch piece of paper, and rule off a 6-inch column. Use that column to take your notes.

2.   Reduce. In the remaining 2-inch column, reduce the main points to a few words or phrases. These are called *cues* or *flags.*

3.   Recite. Looking at both your original notes and the flags in the 2-inch column, recite the main ideas you recorded.

4.   Reflect on the relationships between the main ideas and the flags.

5.   Review, using only the flags. Repeat the process from step 2 for any points that you have difficulty remembering.

MASTERING THE TEXTBOOK

It is important to know how to master textbook information in order to be intellectually prepared for an exam. If you're having difficulty distilling knowledge from your textbook, try the *OK 4R* method: *overview, key ideas, read, recall, reflect,* and *review.*

1.   Overview. Take a look at the portion of your textbook you're trying to master, for example, a chapter or a main section within a chapter. Read the first and last paragraphs. Look at the headings.

2.   Key ideas. Look for the key ideas. Separate the key ideas from any examples. Do not spend a great deal of time reading examples. Convert the key ideas to questions. For example, if the key idea is about the characteristics of schizophrenia, convert that to the question "What are the chief characteristics of schizophrenia?"

3. Read. When you have converted a key idea to a question, read to find the answer to that question and to prove the key point. Continue to ask yourself as you read, "What is the main point?" Do not wait until you're through with the chapter to say, "What is this all about?"

4. Recall the overview, the key ideas and questions, and the answers you found. Now go back and underline and take notes. This will help you avoid over-underlining, which is meaningless.   .

5. Reflect on how new key ideas relate to the old ones that you already know. Think of examples to illustrate the points you have learned.

6. Review the sequence and flow of the main ideas.

MEMORIZING

In preparing for any examination, there are some things you simply have to sit down and memorize. For a nursing examination, they might include:

- *Basic facts:* anatomy (e.g., cranial nerves, layers of muscles), biology (e.g., parts of the cell), nutrition (e.g., sources and effects of vitamins)
- *Nursing history:* key events, dates, places, persons
- *Technical terms and terminology:* types of fractures, insulins, or contraceptive devices, for instance
- *Symbols and abbreviations,* such as those used in charting (c̄, s̄, stat, PRN, ō) SOB, MS, BID
- *Formulas:* chemical formulas, formulas for converting from Centigrade to Fahrenheit, formulas for calculating IV drops per minute

• *Tables:* comparing and contrasting alkalosis and acidosis, hyperglycemia and hypoglycemia, stages of grief, Erikson's stages of growth and development, schedules of immunizations, therapeutic and lethal doses

Memorization Guidelines

1. Think of the content as important.
2. Begin with the intention of remembering, not just reading, the material.
3. Have confidence in your ability to remember.
4. Let go of unsuccessful study patterns, and experiment with new and different ways of studying.
5. Select a time of day and place where you study the best. Apply your time-management procedures as you would for any kind of studying, for example, mastering a portion of your textbook.
6. Eliminate interruptions.
7. Understand the material before you try to memorize it. If you try to learn something that is nonsensical or that you do not understand, it is difficult to retain and recall the information.
8. Associate new information with what you already know.
9. Assign priorities to, and rank-order, what you need to remember the most.
10. Group related points into packets of information.
11. Use and repeat new material. Repetition—overstudying—is extremely important in retaining material. Research has shown a high rate of failure to recall material soon after it's learned. Repetition counters that tendency.
12. Make mistakes work for you.
13. Use mnemonic devices to jog your memory. For example, you might use "On Old Olympus's Towering Tops a Finn and a German Viewed Some Hops" to help you memorize the twelve cranial nerves.

Additional Items

- *Break the information down into small, basic units.*
  Research has shown that people can retain only seven
  items, plus or minus two, in short-term memory. If
  you can break up a long list into smaller units, it will
  be easier to remember. The traditional "Alphabet
  Song" is a good example; the letters are broken down
  into units of one to four letters each: AB, CD, EFG, HI,
  etc.

- *Create some kind of internal organization.* It's easier
  to remember something that has a meaningful structure than something that is random or abstract. Here
  are some ways to organize:
  * Look for a natural hierarchy in the material: What is
    the most important thing? What builds on what?
  * Make up a story or a narrative chain to relate events
    to one another.
  * Find some kind of external organization between
    new information and that information you already
    know. Information is useless if it's not properly cat-
    alogued.

- Oldest mnemonic device is *loci,* used by Greek and
  Roman orators. Imagine that the various words to be
  learned are located at different physical locations (*loci*
  means "points" in Latin). To recall the words, visualize a location, such as the front door to your house,
  and discover the word that you've associated with it.

- Rhyme is another mnemonic device. Common examples include:
  * *i* before *e* except after *c*
  * the alphabet song
  * 30 days hath September, April, June, and November.
    All the rest have 31, except the second month,
    which has 28, and Leap Year gives it 29.

- Association gives meaning to abstract words, phrases,
  or lists.

Those who have taken piano lessons may have learned to associate the phrase "Every Good Boy Does Fine" with the notes on the lines of the treble clef in music, which associates thoughts to places. But thoughts can also be associated or linked to one another. To learn a list of ten items, begin by creating an image of the first item. Say the first item is an orange. Picture an orange in your mind's eye. The second item is a wheelbarrow. Now create an image that ties the orange to the wheelbarrow: for example, a gigantic orange with handles like a wheelbarrow, or a wheelbarrow filled with oranges. Say the third item is a book. To link it to the wheelbarrow, you might picture a book about wheelbarrows or a book with handles being pushed along like a wheelbarrow. Continue down the list.

5

How to Take Tests

UNDERSTANDING TEST CONSTRUCTION

When you have information about the guidelines used to prepare multiple-choice items, you can anticipate what the structure and the format of the questions may be. This should help reduce your test-taking anxiety.

Items are written so they focus on an important concept or idea. Each item is structured around one central idea or problem that is clearly presented in the stem and to which all options relate in the same way. Each item has one and only one correct (best) answer. The language used is simple, direct, and free of ambiguity. The examinee is expected to arrive at the answer from information provided in the material, *not* from having answered correctly a previous question in the set. Distractors in one question are not meant to provide clues for answering any other question in the set. To test factual knowledge, the item writer does not dress up the item to appear otherwise. To test critical thinking, the item writer makes sure the item cannot be answered on the basis of factual information alone. To make an item a difficult one, the item writer makes certain it requires sophisticated reasoning or understanding of a high-level concept, not obscure or esoteric knowledge. Double negatives are rarely used.

The Stem

The stem may be written as a question, as an incomplete statement to be completed by the options, or as a complete statement of a problem to be solved. The stem is written so the examinee's task is clearly defined and so the examinee has all the information needed to understand the item's intent.

Distractors

The distractors are chosen so that incorrectness is not the sole criterion. Good distractors might include the following:

1. Common misconceptions and common errors.
2. A statement that itself is true but does not satisfy the requirement of the problem.
3. A statement that is either too broad or too narrow for the requirement of the problem.
4. A carefully worded incorrect statement that may sound plausible to the uninformed.

The Wording of Options

Options are phrased so they maintain a similar relationship to the thought in the stem and state their idea clearly and concisely. Each option has the same similarity to the stem as the correct answer—in wording or in grammatical construction. Correct answers usually avoid textbookish wording. They also are written so they are not consistently longer than the distractors. Distractors are written with as much care and precision as the correct answer so that all alternatives are equally attractive to an examinee who guesses. Giveaways in the distractors—for example, "always," "only," "every," "all," "never"—may be avoided, since sophisticated examinees can recognize that statements containing these terms are seldom universally true. Words with unfavorable connotations are *not* used if they would contrast sharply with words having favorable connotations in the stem, and vice versa. When the stem asks for an evaluation—for example, "best" or "most"—the examinee is required to identify "the best" or "the most" of several options rather than to distinguish what is correct from what is incorrect.

STRATEGIES FOR TAKING MULTIPLE-CHOICE TESTS

1. Skim the test for an overview of intent, scope, and pattern, that is, for trivial detail *versus* basic principles, memorization *versus* application, abstract *versus* concrete situations.
2. Use deductive reasoning.
3. Be aware of *absurd* options. By a process of elimination, weed out absurd, unsound, unreasonable options or those that do not fit. Know how to choose between options that sound *similar;* that is, choose the one that encompasses the others. Know how to focus in on *conflicting* options: either one or neither is the correct answer, never both.
4. Stem–option resemblance: The best answer will be a direct repetition in the option as it relates to and resembles the stem, or there will be an *associative* connection between the stem and the option.
5. Cue-using strategies: Learn how to obtain cues from other options to assist you in selecting the best answers. If there is a cue to specific detail, then the more specific the stem, the more information is needed; therefore, look for the detailed answer. *Key words:* Be aware of specific determiners as to the best answer. Be aware of *grammatical* cues.
6. Mentally anticipate what the answer might be, then

check the options for what comes closest to your guess. Suspend making a choice until you have read all the options. The most plausible decoys may be listed first. And although all options may be true, only one of them is best.

7. Relate options to the question to fit their requirement. Does the question ask for a reason?

8. The correct statement may be the wrong answer (for instance, when the stem asks for the option that *doesn't* fit).

9. Compare one option against the others when several seem right. Find what makes them *different*. For example, if both seem right but one focuses on feelings rather than facts, choose the one that deals with feelings if it's a question on interpersonal relations. When two or more look correct, choose the *encompassing* option as the best choice. Look for the "umbrella" example as the best answer. For instance: Which of the following cities are in the State of New York? (A) Syracuse; (B) Rome; (C) Albany; (D) All of the above; (E) None of the above. The correct answer is D. If you know that both Syracuse and Albany are in New York, then you know that the answer must include at least two of the cities; therefore, in this option set the answer has to be "all of the above."

10. A statement is true only if it is true *without* exception. For example, the statement "Families with more children are poorer than families with fewer children" cannot be true because there are exceptions. Therefore, the answer is "false."

11. Budget your time. For example, complete two questions per minute if there are 120 questions in a 2-hour test. Guess at or leave out difficult questions, and note down which ones. Use any leftover time to take another look at those and to reconsider answers, checking for errors.

12. Read instructions carefully. You must understand what is wanted. Never assume that directions for

one section will apply in other sections; never assume that all questions even in the same sections will ask you the same kind of thing. For example, one time the directions may say "Which of the following is *least* important?" Another time they may ask for the *"most* important."

13. Answer only what is asked about, not what you think should be asked about.

14. Read the questions slowly and carefully; don't jump to conclusions. Keep the focus of the question in mind.

15. Focus on the demands of the question. Look for *key* words, such as "distinguish," "describe," "compare," "if," "same as," "similar to," "illustrate," "summarize," "opposite of." Watch for units of measurement, such as, time, amount, dose.

16. Consider the level of sophistication of the test. Don't read into questions or answers too deeply.

17. Know the purpose of the exam and the intent of the item-writer. The purpose of the licensure exam is to measure safe, *not* expert, performance; practitioner's, *not* specialist's, knowledge and behaviors; nursing knowledge and skills, *not* physician's knowledge and skills.

18. Maintain a positive, open attitude: "I may not know the answer but I can figure it out." The unfamiliar points may not be essential for determining the best answers.

19. Attempt every question. Do not avoid complicated-looking questions.

20. Think about the best answer. Do not rely on intuition.

21. Don't misread or overlook *key* words or phrases, such as "not," "except," "all," "only," "none."

22. Be clear on the directions before you start. Test items cause problems when they are complex due to length of the stem or the options, or to key words, or to levels of sophistication.

HOW AND WHEN TO GUESS

1. Blind versus informed guessing. *Blind guessing* involves material that is completely unfamiliar. *Informed guessing* means you *eliminate* the absurd options and then *guess on the basis of familiarity.*

2. Anticipate characteristics that should be present in a correct option before reading the options. And read *all* the options before selecting the correct one. Relate each option to the stem.

3. Reason actively. Don't just sit and wait for the right answer to pop out. Ask yourself: What is the main point of the question? What are the key terms? What is my best guess? What are the elements of this question? What *concepts* apply? What can I draw on from my *experience* that is relevant to this question? What kind of answer is needed here? Can I *rephrase* the question? Can I *break it down* into parts?

4. Make a question more concrete by translating and *substituting* terms to simplify the question. Use a *synonym* to make sense of a question. Substitute an *illustration*, a *specific situation*, an *example*, or an abstract term to help you think through a problem.

5. Break the question down into manageable parts. Knowing part of an answer may provide clues to the best answer.

6. Look for cues and information from *other* questions to help you choose a particular answer.

7. Ignore irrelevant information and get to the main point of a question. Don't get too preoccupied with the content or meaning of a case description before you know what the question is asking for. Use logic and common sense whenever possible.

Clues in the Construction of the Test

1. Specific determiners. Options with the words "all," "none," "always," "must," or "never" are seldom the correct options.
2. Look for a repeat of a stem word in one of the options.
3. The implied definition of a key word in the stem may be found in one of the responses.
4. Possible uniformity in the position of correct answers. They tend *not* to be the first or the last option, often clustering in the center.
5. The best answers are grammatically correct and consistent with the stem.
6. When questions involve numbers, dates, or quantities, the correct response is often in the mid-range of chronology or size rather than one of the extremes of the option set.
7. Exceptionally long or short options may have a pattern of being obviously correct or obviously wrong.
8. Obvious distractors may include flippant, humorous, or absolutely unreasonable responses.
9. Options with qualifying words such as "usually," "frequently," "some," "sometimes," "generally," "often," or "seldom" tend to be the better responses.
10. A correct response is often broader, more generally applicable, and more comprehensive than the other choices.
11. When options overlap, the choice that encompasses the others should be selected.
12. Overly technical, unfamiliar language is rarely included in the correct responses.
13. Correct responses usually do not contain emotionally charged words, such as "idiot," or "stupid."

6
Guidelines
for Taking the
NCLEX-RN Exam

TRENDS IN TEST DESIGN

Nursing tests are changing to include questions that test not only knowledge but the following intellectual abilities, which are based on a classification developed by test experts Benjamin Bloom and David Kratwohl.

Comprehension: Recall and Understanding

a. Translation: the ability to express an idea in a form different from what is given.

b. Interpretation: the ability to explain how one idea relates to another.

c. Extrapolation: the ability to project and predict a trend from given information.

Application: the ability to appropriately use principles, abstractions, and rules in specific situations.

Analysis: the ability to identify component parts.

Synthesis: the ability to put elements and parts together to form a new whole.

Evaluation: the ability to assess results and make value judgments.

The NCLEX exam has moved away from being a test of medical knowledge to being a test of nursing behaviors, that is, the five steps of the nursing process. In the past, items were designed to test simple recall; now they test primarily *application* and *analysis* of knowledge, so mere rote memorization of facts is of little help. In the past, some of the items on the RN licensure exam dealt with the ideal—nursing as it should be. The trend now is for questions to measure the beginning practitioner's ability to practice in today's actual nursing world, in all clinical areas and at the basic entry level. Thus, the exam is more realistic and based on actual standards of nursing practice.

STRUCTURE AND FORMAT OF THE NCLEX-RN EXAM*

The following sections contain the most current information about the current RN licensure.

Exam Questions Test for Safe, Effective Nursing Practice

The following outline of categories of safe, effective practice is from a study by Angeline Jacobs and others, entitled *Critical Requirements for Safe/Effective Nursing Practice* and published in 1978 by the American Nurses' Association.* The test plan reflects nursing practice as identified in 2,000 critical incidents collected and analyzed for this study as well as 222 activities identified in the job analysis of what

---

*Adapted from *Practice Questions & Answers for NCLEX-RN*. Review for Nurses Tapes, Inc., San Francisco, CA: 1989, pp. 35–42.

an entry level nurse does in a study by Michael Kane and others. Nursing behaviors tested in the exam are derived from these research studies on the validity of the State Board Test Pool Examination, which identified behaviors relevant to current nursing practice in each of the five clinical specialties.

1. Exercises professional prerogatives based on clinical judgment.
   a. Adapts care to individual patient needs.
   b. Fulfills responsibility to patient and others despite difficulty.
   c. Challenges inappropriate orders and decisions by medical and other professional staff.
   d. Acts as patient advocate in obtaining appropriate medical, psychiatric, or other help.
   e. Recognizes own limitations and errors.
   f. Analyzes and adjusts own or staff reactions in order to maintain therapeutic relationship with patient.

2. Promotes patient's ability to cope with immediate, long-range, or potential health-related change.
   a. Provides health care instruction or information to patient, family, or significant others.
   b. Encourages patient or family to make decisions about accepting care or adhering to treatment regime.
   c. Helps patient recognize and deal with psychological stress.
   d. Avoids creating or increasing anxiety or stress.
   e. Conveys and invites acceptance, respect, and trust.
   f. Facilitates relationship of family, staff, or significant others with patient.

Sources: Literature from National Council of State Boards of Nursing; A new licensing exam for nurses, *American Journal of Nursing* (4) (April 1980): 723–725. Report of study conducted by the American College Testing Program for the National Council of State Boards of Nursing, Inc., 1986: *A Study of Nursing Practice and Role Delineation of Entry Level Performance of Registered Nurses.*

g. Stimulates and remotivates patient, or enables him or her to achieve self-care and independence.

3. Helps maintain patient comfort and normal body functions.
   a. Keeps patient clean and comfortable.
   b. Helps patient maintain or regain normal body functions.

4. Takes precautionary and preventive measures in giving patient care.
   a. Prevents infection.
   b. Protects skin and mucous membranes from injurious materials.
   c. Uses positioning or exercise to prevent injury or the complications of immobility.
   d. Avoids using injurious technique in administering and managing intrusive or other potentially traumatic treatments.
   e. Protects patient from falls or other contact injuries.
   f. Maintains surveillance of patient's activities.
   g. Reduces or removes environmental hazards.

5. Checks, compares, verifies, monitors, and follows up medication and treatment processes.
   a. Checks correctness, condition, and safety of medication being prepared.
   b. Ensures that correct medication or care is given to the right patient and that patient takes or receives it.
   c. Adheres to schedule in giving medication, treatment, or test.
   d. Administers medication by correct route, rate, or mode.
   e. Checks patient's readiness for medication, treatment, surgery, or other care.
   f. Checks to ensure that tests or measurements are done correctly.
   g. Monitors ongoing infusions and inhalations.
   h. Checks for and interprets effect of medication,

treatment, or care, and takes corrective action if necessary.

6. Interprets symptom complex and intervenes appropriately.
   a. Checks patient's condition or status.
   b. Remains objective, further investigates, or verifies patient's complaint or problem.
   c. Uses alarms and signals on automatic equipment as adjunct to personal assessment.
   d. Observes and correctly assesses signs of anxiety or behavioral stress.
   e. Observes and correctly assesses physical signs, symptoms, or findings, and intervenes appropriately.
   f. Correctly assesses severity or priority of patient's condition, and gives or obtains necessary care.

7. Responds to emergencies.
   a. Anticipates need for crisis care.
   b. Takes instant, correct action in emergency situations.
   c. Maintains calm and efficient approach under pressure.
   d. Assumes leadership role in crisis situation when necessary.

8. Obtains, records, and exchanges information on behalf of the patient.
   a. Checks data sources for orders and other information about patient.
   b. Obtains information from patient and family.
   c. Transcribes or records information on chart, Kardex, or other information system.
   d. Exchanges information with nursing staff and other departments.
   e. Exchanges information with medical staff.

9. Utilizes patient-care planning.
   a. Develops and modifies patient care plan.
   b. Implements patient care plan.

   10. Teaches and supervises other staff.
      a. Teaches correct principles, procedures, and techniques of patient care.
      b. Supervises and checks the work of staff for whom she or he is responsible.

Exam Questions Test Application and Analysis

About 80% of the items test two levels of cognitive knowledge (as described by Benjamin Bloom):

* *Application:* The use of abstractions in particular or concrete situations. They may be in the form of general ideas, rules, procedures, or general methods. The abstractions may also be technical principles, ideas, and theories that need to be remembered and applied.
* *Analysis:* The breakdown of the whole into constituent parts or elements so that a rank priority of ideas can emerge and relationships between ideas can be made clear.

Recall and comprehension levels (understanding) will *not* be emphasized.

Categories of Nursing Knowledge

* Normal growth and development through the life cycle.
  Recommendation: Review theories of growth and development by Duvall, Sullivan, Piaget, Freud, and Erikson.
* Basic human needs.
  Recommendation: Review Maslow and Havighurst.
* Coping mechanisms used by individuals.
  Recommendation: Review most common adaptive behaviors, e.g., blocking, compensation, denial, displace-

ment, fixation, identification, introjection, projection, rationalization, reaction formation, regression, repression, sublimation, substitution, suppression, undoing.

- Common health problems (actual or potential) in the major health areas and based on current morbidity studies.
  Recommendation: Review ten most common diseases, disorders, and causes of death.

- Variations in health needs as affected by age, sex, culture, ethnicity, and religion.
  Recommendation: Be aware of food preferences and dietary restrictions; belief systems about causes of illness, methods of treatment, concept of death, concept of time; kinship structure and roles of the male, the female, and the extended family; ethnic variations in susceptibility to certain diseases.

- Nursing goals and interventions to assist individuals in maintaining life and health, coping with health problems, and/or recovering from the effects of injury or disease.
  Recommendation: Review nursing priorities for patients in life-threatening situations, health teaching and health maintenance situations, and rehabilitation situations.

Concepts Relevant to Nursing Practice

- Management.
- Accountability.
  Recommendation: Review major legal and ethical issues, areas of nursing responsibilities, and standards of nursing practice.
- Life cycle.
  Recommendation: Review major health concerns, problems, and nursing care during birth, childhood, school age, adolescence, young adult and reproductive years, middle age, and older adult and geriatric years.

- Client environment.
  Recommendation: Review measures to protect from harm against airborne irritants, cold, and heat; review approaches to eliminate environmental discomforts, such as odors, noise, poor ventilation, dust; know safety hazards; review measures to maintain environmental order and cleanliness.

Categories of Client Needs

The test items emphasize four categories of client needs with 17 subcategories of activities designed to meet these needs.

- About half of the items (42–48%) will emphasize meeting the clients' physical needs in actual or potential life-threatening, chronic, recurring *Physiological* conditions; and clients who are at risk for complications or untoward effects of treatment. Subcategories include:
    1. *Physiological Adaptation:* meeting acute physical needs.
    2. *Reduction of Risk Potential:* monitoring clients at risk.
    3. *Mobility:* assisting clients with mobility needs.
    4. *Comfort:* controlling pain.
    5. *Provision of Basic Care:* performing routine nursing activities.
- *Safe, Effective Care Environment* is the second highest category (25–31%) of emphasis. Subcategories include:
    1. *Coordinated Care:* staff development, collaboration
    2. *Quality Assurance and Safety.*
    3. *Goal-Oriented Care:* planning, managing client care.
    4. *Environmental Safety:* protecting the client.
    5. *Preparation for Treatments and Procedures:* preparing clients for procedures.

6. *Safe and Effective Treatments and Procedures:* ensuring safety during the procedures.
- The next highest (12–18%) category of emphasis (*Health Promotion and Maintenance*) includes these subcategories:
    1. *Continued Growth and Development Throughout the Life Cycle:* meeting client needs related to parenting.
    2. *Self-Care:* assisting clients with self-care.
    3. *Support Systems:* supporting client's family.
    4. *Prevention and Early Treatment of Disease:* immunizing/screening.
- Lastly 9–15% of the items will be on *Psychosocial* integrity, with a focus on stress and crisis related situations throughout the life cycle. Subcategories include:
    1. *Psychosocial Adaptation:* meeting acute emotional and behavioral needs.
    2. *Coping/Adaptation:* helping clients to cope with stress.

The 5-Step Nursing Process Applied to Client Situations

The following five specific kinds of nursing behaviors measured on the NCLEX-RN are given equal weight (15% to 25%) in all of the client situations listed above, in all stages of the life cycle.

1. *Assessment:* ability to assess.
2. *Analysis:* ability to analyze data and identify specific needs.
3. *Planning:* ability to plan and set goals.
4. *Implementation:* ability to implement specific actions.
5. *Evaluation:* ability to evaluate outcome.

Sample Questions

Examples of questions that focus on specific nursing behaviors (that is, aspects of the five steps of the nursing process) are:

1. *Assessment* (This question is also an example of shared decision-making by both client and nurse.)

   A multigravida client in labor is admitted to the maternity unit. What information does the nurse need in order to evaluate the status of the client's labor?
   A. Blood pressure.
   B. FHR.
   C. Contour of abdomen.
   D. Duration, frequency, and intervals of contractions.

   Comment: You need to know the relative importance of the signs and symptoms of labor in order to assess the status of labor when all the signs are correct. In this case, *D* is the most important. There is a need for interaction between the nurse and client to assess the client's progress in labor.

2. *Analysis*

   A 30-year-old man with diabetes, who has previously been stabilized on insulin, calls the emergency room to relate that although his urine is negative for sugar and acetone, he feels as if he is about to pass out. He reports that he has been eating three regular meals a day and taking his insulin as directed. What would be a valid interpretation of his current condition?
   A. He is not physically active enough.
   B. He needs to change his insulin dose.
   C. He has low blood sugar.
   D. His insulin level is high.

   Comment: In order to select *C* as the best answer,

you need not only to understand diabetes, but also to assess the symptoms and to interpret them correctly.

3. *Planning*

A comatose client is admitted to the hospital. Which of the following nursing goals would be of prime importance at the outset?
A. Establish a flexible visiting schedule so that his relatives can watch him closely.
B. Include the family in his immediate physical care.
C. Provide consistency of care by assigning the same nursing personnel to him.
D. Place him in a room where you can closely monitor his condition from the nursing station.

Comment: To choose the best response, *D,* you need to analyze the situation correctly and apply that knowledge in planning a strategy to achieve the goal of providing close observation of the client's condition.

4. *Implementation* (This question is also an example of a situation where the nurse makes the decisions.)

An emaciated-looking patient with anorexia nervosa is admitted to the mental health unit. She refuses to eat lunch when it is served, just as she has refused most meals at home. What can the nurse say that would be most effective in encouraging her to eat?
A. "You will have to eat if you do not want us to tube-feed you."
B. "Here is a small sandwich. I will sit with you to keep you company while you eat."
C. "It is important that you eat your meals, as it is part of your therapy to help you gain weight."
D. "Aren't you hungry? It is a long time before you can eat dinner if you don't eat your lunch."

Comment: B is the best nursing action, to provide for

the basic need for nutrition when the client's psychological condition prevents her from taking care of her own physiological need for food.

5. *Evaluation* (This question is also an example of a situation where the client makes the decisions.)

An obese man began his weight loss program after Christmas. The plan was for him to lose a minimum of 10 pounds a month. By February 1, he had lost 15 pounds. What action should the nurse take at this time?
A. Praise him for his results and ask him if he would like to set the next goal at 15 pounds.
B. Refer him to the dietician to regulate his weight loss.
C. Encourage him to lose even more weight since he is doing so well.
D. Ask him why he lost more weight than planned.

Comment: The weight loss is controlled by the client, with the nurse providing needed support and encouragement. Here, the best answer is *A* because it measures the results (15 pounds) against the goal (10 pounds) and works with the client to change the goal appropriately.

Summary

Based on the above discussion of the established percentage of the number of test items, the following is a sample test plan showing the relative emphasis (number of test questions) on (1) specific nursing behaviors and (2) health needs of clients.

Specific Nursing Behaviors

Nursing Behaviors Tested	Percentage of Test Items Related to Specific Behaviors
Assessment	15–25%
Analysis	15–25
Planning	15–25
Implementation	15–25
Evaluation	15–25

Categories of Health Needs of Clients

Client Need	Percentage of Test Items
Physiological Integrity	42–48%
Safe, Effective Care Environment	25–31
Health Promotion and Maintenance	12–18
Psychosocial Integrity	9–15

Practical Exercises for Improving Test Performance

This chapter presents simple exercises you can practice by yourself to greatly improve your test-taking skills. They will:

1. Promote relaxation and an open mind
2. Give affirmation
3. Calm the mind
4. Recall pleasure in learning
5. Promote rhythmic breathing
6. Improve concentration
7. Aid memory
8. Accentuate the positive self-image of a successful learner

Through sequential steps in visualization it is possible to improve *concentration*, enhance mental abilities, and develop a photographic or visual *memory*.

The simple, sequential exercises that follow have helped many; they can work for you. They can help you increase your learning potential and feel good while doing it. You can fulfill your learning potential by learning how to ease stress, and you can open your mind to expand your awareness.

Heightened achievement will follow increased awareness. These exercises are designed to *strengthen concentration and memory* and thus to accelerate the learning of factual material.

Physical Relaxation (Progressive Relaxation)

Objective.   This exercise is a preliminary one that must be practiced at least a week before starting any memory training. Practice regularly to familiarize yourself with the techniques for ridding your body of tension and fatigue—a necessary first step to opening yourself up to learning. This exercise will help your mind to be *active, stay alert,* and *concentrate better.*

Technique.

1. Find a comfortable place where you will not be interrupted. Choose a very comfortable position, either sitting in a chair or lying on a couch or on the floor.
2. Loosen constrictive clothing.
3. Become aware of how your bones and muscles make contact with the chair, couch, or floor.
4. Close your eyes.
5. Take in a slow, deep breath.
6. Exhale. As you do so, feel the tension leaving your body. Tell yourself to let go, to relax.
7. Take in a second breath, very slowly and deeply.
8. Exhale. Feel the tension floating away with the breath.
9. Take in a third slow, deep breath.
10. Exhale. Allow more tension to leave until you are calm and peaceful.
11. Now, one at a time, tense up each of your muscles, going from toes to head, in the following order: toes, feet, ankles, lower leg, knee, upper leg, buttocks, lower back, abdomen, chest, shoulders, back, upper arm, elbow, lower arm, wrist, hands, neck, jaw, lips, tongue, teeth, throat, cheeks, eyes, forehead, scalp.

Do this until your entire body is tense.

12. Maintain the tension for several seconds.

13. Let a wave of relaxation go through your body, from head to toe.

14. Repeat this tensing and relaxing *three* times. During each cycle, count slowly to 15.

Psychological Relaxation (Visualization)

Objective.   Many people find it is easier to relax using mental imagery rather than progressive physical tensing and relaxing. If that is your preference, then do the following exercise instead.

Technique.

1. Make yourself as comfortable as possible—sit in a chair or lie down on a couch or the floor.

2. Loosen tight clothing.

3. Close your eyes.

4. Take several slow, deep, even breaths. As you breathe easily and deeply, visualize the following: Project yourself to the seventh floor of a building. See the walls painted a vivid, warm *red.* Walk down this red hallway to the end, where you arrive at the top of a "down" escalator painted silver. See the escalator as smooth, noiseless, and completely secure and dependable. Step on the escalator and feel yourself beginning to glide down. Your hands are on the rails and you descend without any sound—very slowly, very safely, very securely. As you ride down, you feel yourself unwinding and relaxing, unwinding and relaxing.

5. Take a deep breath. As you exhale, say the number "seven" several times. Visualize a large number seven standing out against the vivid red walls of the seventh floor. The red color seems to float past you as you continue your relaxing ride down. You have now reached the sixth floor. Get off the escalator and see the number six painted on the bright *orange* walls of the sixth floor. Surrounded by this bright orange color, walk to the head of the next "down" escalator and step on it. Again, glide slowly downward.

6. Take a deep breath. As you exhale, repeat the number "six" several times and see the pleasant orange walls all around you. Feel yourself unwinding and relaxing as you smoothly ride down to a still more restful and pleasant spot. You have now reached the fifth floor. See the fifth floor sign, and notice the delightful, golden *yellow* walls. Get off the escalator and walk through this corridor of yellow to the next "down" escalator.

7. Take a deep breath, and while exhaling visualize the number "five." Mentally repeat "five" several times while enjoying the beautiful, joyous, golden yellow. Get on the next escalator and continue to float downward. Feel how comfortable you are, how easy, as you let yourself go and simply enjoy the colors.

8. Take a deep breath, and as you exhale read the number "four" sign and notice the restful, lush, emerald *green* walls. Get off the escalator on the fourth floor, and walk through this clear, emerald green hallway to the next "down" escalator.

9. Take a deep breath as you step onto the escalator and begin once again to glide downward, smoothly and easily, exhaling as you read the number "three" and arrive at a still more pleasant and relaxing area of soft and restful *blue*. Step off the escalator, walk through the soft blue corridor to the next "down" escalator.

10. Take the escalator to the second floor. See the second-floor sign, and see the rich *purple* walls. Get off the escalator.

11. Take a deep breath, and while exhaling visualize the number two. Mentally repeat "two" several times. Sense the rich purple all around you, and feel how wonderfully comfortable and relaxed you are. Move through this purple onto the next "down" escalator.

As you descend, see the first-floor sign, notice that the main floor is a luminous *violet* color. The escalator glides softly downward. Get off at the first floor.

12. Take a deep breath, and while exhaling visualize the number one and repeat "one" several times. Enjoy the luminous violet all around you. You have now achieved a state of deep relaxation. You are completely rested, healthy, and relaxed. You have reached your main inner space. Here you can easily connect in your mind with other areas of awareness. Remain in this state of complete relaxation and continue to breath deeply. You are completely relaxed. (This is an ideal time to practice some of the positive self-affirmations to be described next.)

13. To return from this main inner space, count from one to three. On the count of three, open your eyes and feel alert, centered, refreshed, and free of all tensions.

Affirming Your Ability to Learn

Objective.   Affirmations should be performed when you are relaxed and at peace. Thus they usually *follow* a relaxation exercise. Instead of the following phrases you can make up your own short, rhythmic phrases to fit your needs. Try using rhyme or alliteration—for example, "I feel calm under a palm," or "My mind is marvelous and masterful."

Technique.   With your eyes closed, repeat silently—four times—any one of the following phrases.

I can do it!

I can reach my goal.

Learning is something I enjoy.

Learning is easy for me.

It is easy to remember.

My mind is working efficiently.

I can work effectively.

I am truly calm.

Before tests:

I can remember what I want to.

I *will* remember what is important.

I can recognize the best answer when I need to.

I am truly confident.

My memory is working, my mind is alert.

Calming Your Mind—Visualization

Objective.   To calm your mind and eliminate tensions and worries, practice visualizing peaceful scenes from nature. Through sequential visualization steps you can *improve your concentration, enhance your mental abilities, stimulate your memory,* and *focus your mind.*

Technique.   Visualize a place that has a relaxing effect on you, such as a lake, a mountain, a ski slope, woods, or a beach. For example:

Imagine yourself on a wide, sandy beach.

Feel the warmth of the sun as you stretch out on the sand.

Picture yourself strolling along the surf's edge.

Feel the sand between your toes as you walk.

Feel the gentle surf washing over your feet.

Enjoy the gentle breeze blowing through your hair— blowing away your cares and concerns.

Listen to the distant calls of the seagulls.

Look up and see how blue the sky is. See the one or two billowy white clouds floating slowly by.

See the water—turquoise and clear and sparkling.

See the sparkling pattern the sun is making on the water.

Feel how all is peaceful and calm.

Stay with the scene, savor it as much as possible.

Calming Your Mind—Color Encounters

Objective.   This visualization exercise is another way to calm your mind.

Technique.   Take a comfortable position, close your eyes and raise them slightly upward. Take a deep breath through your nose and, while exhaling slowly, feel a wave of warm relaxation slowly flowing over your entire body, from your toes to your head. Use your preferred relaxation method to reach a comfortable state of relaxation. One by one you will visualize dots of colored light suspended in space a short distance from you, and see them grow larger and larger, come closer and closer, then become paler and paler and gradually float off into space.

1. Visualize a dot of *red* light in front of you—bright, vivid, red light. See it becoming larger and larger. See the red light coming closer and closer. Watch how the red light grows paler and paler and slowly begins to fade into the distance.
2. Next picture an *orange* dot of light. Imagine the rich orange light coming closer and getting bigger and bigger like a spotlight. See the orange light fading, getting paler and paler and slowly becoming like a cloud of light as it fades into the distance.
3. Now, visualize a *yellow* dot of light. See how—just like a beam of a spotlight—it comes closer and closer, getting bigger and brighter. Bask in this golden circle of yellow light for a minute. Then see the light gradually get paler and paler and float away.
4. Now look at a *green* dot—a clear, emerald green dot of light. Watch it come closer and closer until all you

see is pure emerald green. Then see the green light fade, becoming paler as it disappears from sight.

5. Visualize a *soft blue* dot of light. See the blue light coming closer and closer, getting bigger and bigger and encircling you, until it totally embraces you. Let it lift you gently up as it gets paler and paler until it forms a buoyant, white cloud of light.

6. Imagine yourself floating up into the sky on this wonderful cloud of *white* light. Become aware of other clouds as you float past them. Enjoy the tranquil feeling of peace and happiness throughout your body. You feel relaxed, calm, healthy, competent. Whenever you wish, you can remember this feeling. You can remember the centered, calm feeling before an exam when it will help you.

7. Now gently start to come back. Feel yourself slowly returning to your usual surroundings and to a more aware self. Slowly open your eyes. Take several breaths, stretch, and turn on all your body switches. You feel centered and rested.

Waking Dream—Visualization

Objective. This exercise combines relaxation and visualization to *open the creative part of your mind* and help you *feel peaceful and serene.*

Technique. Take a comfortable position. Close your eyes and raise them slightly upward. Take a deep breath through your nose and, while exhaling slowly, feel a warm wave of relaxation slowly flow over your entire body, from your toes to your head. Use your preferred relaxation method to reach a state of relaxation.

Imagine yourself walking along a winding path in a lush, green, wooded area; ahead of you is a small, grassy hill. Slowly and easily start climbing the hill. Notice the wildflowers nestled in the long grass along the path. Hear the pebbles crunch as you walk over them. Pause as you reach the top of the hill. At the bottom of this hill you can see a small, winding stream. Slowly descend the hill towards the stream. Feel the cool, soft grass under your feet. Follow the path sloping down the hill to level ground and move to the edge of the stream. Look along the bank and see the slender willows bending over the water. See the thick, brown mud of the banks. Watch the sunlight reflecting in the cool, clear water as it flows along. As you reach the edge of the stream, notice a raft.

See how this raft is made of thick wood. See its surface polished smooth and blanketed with soft, cushiony moss. You are aware that this is a safe and secure raft. Climb on the raft. Push it away from shore, and settle back to feel a wave of warm relaxation envelop you as you float along.

Feel the gentle rise and fall of the waves. Become aware of the easy rocking motion as you slowly drift along. Listen to the gentle lapping of the water against the raft. Enjoy total relaxation as you float downstream toward a small tunnel, a familiar, safe tunnel where for a while you can be shaded from the sun. As you enter the tunnel, see the sparkling water at the other end. This is a dream tunnel. As you enter the comfortable darkness of the tunnel, let yourself dream. Look into the darkness. Take your time, and let whatever will, come and play itself out in your mind.

As you pass out of the tunnel, feel yourself being bathed in warm, bright sunshine. Feel that sunlight bringing you energy and happiness.

Smell the fresh country scents of stream and grass as a gentle breeze passes over you. Open all your senses. Fill all your pores with the nature around you. Look over the side of the raft and see the many different-colored fish swimming by. Notice the various colors and shapes as the fish gleam and dart. Then look at the banks and see the leafy branches overhanging the stream. Glimpse the birds moving in the leaves. Then look at the sky above. Feel contentment and serenity as you peacefully drift along, like the small white clouds in the sky, gliding effortlessly, high up in the blue. Feel the quietness around you. Take a moment to think about tranquility, harmony, and peace. Feel the warmth of the sun envelop your body. Become fully aware of being within this experience—the flowing motion of the raft, the warmth, the smells, the sounds as you drift along. Become one with the sensations around you.

Now gently return from this place in your mind: Count from one to five. Slowly become aware of your present surroundings. Feel your body switch on as you slowly open your eyes and look around the room. Stretch and take a few deep breaths. You feel centered and rested.

Recalling the Joy of Learning

Objective. This exercise will enable you to *reexperience the good feelings* that come with *successful learning.*

Technique. Think back to a time when you felt successful in learning something, or when you remembered a particular piece of information. It can be the memory of when you first learned to ride a bike, solved a riddle, or came up with the key missing word in a crossword puzzle. Recall that exhilarating sense of accomplishment when you memorized your part in a school play. Remember when you learned something fascinating.

Relive the complete details of such a positive learning experience. Feel the pleasure again of being successful in learning. What was it like? Who was there? How did you feel? How did you feel in your stomach? in your hands and legs? in your head? Recapture the sense of excitement you had about that learning experience. Enjoy the pleasure of what your mind and memory felt like when it came through for you, when you learned with ease. Hold on to this mind set, this exceptional feeling. Savor it.

Rhythmic Breathing

Objective. This exercise will *slow down* your mind, your body, and your rhythms to the most efficient level by controlling your breathing with a rhythmic pattern.

Technique.

1. Assume a comfortable position in a chair or bed or on a couch. Completely relax your entire body.
2. Close your eyes, and breathe in very slowly, deeply, and evenly through your nose. When you think you have taken in as much air as possible, take in a little more. Pouch out your stomach. Hold your breath for a count of three.
3. Exhale slowly, and pull in your stomach. Exhale as completely as possible. Now try to exhale a little more. As you exhale let a feeling of relaxation sweep over you.
4. Repeat the deep inhalation–exhalation for several minutes, each time taking in a slow, even, deep breath.
5. Now inhale as you count from one to four. Then hold your breath for another count from one to four. Then exhale as you count from one to four again. Finally, pause as you once more count from one to four. Repeat this process four times.
6. Next, slow your in-and-out breathing to a count of six. Repeat this four times.
7. Finally, slow your rhythmic breathing to a count of eight. Repeat four times. For example—breathe in, two, three, four, five, six, seven, eight. Hold it, two, three, four, five, six, seven, eight. Breathe out, two, three, four, five, six, seven, eight. Pause, two, three, four, five, six, seven, eight.

Concentration Exercise 1

Objective.   This exercise will help *focus your concentration.* You will *need* to have a rock handy.

Technique.   First relax in your preferred way.

1. Reach out and take the rock in your hand. Turn it over and over. Examine it. Is it smooth or rough? hard

or porous? Does it have a smell? Does it have a taste?

2. Now relax still more. Close your eyes and imagine that you are very, very small—tiny enough to crawl inside the rock and look around.

3. Now imagine that you *are* the rock. How does it feel? Are you heavy or light? large or small?

4. Now pretend you, the rock, are lying out in a field of grass. Imagine a gentle rain falling on you. How does the rain affect you? Are there any changes in the ground you are lying on?

5. Now imagine that the rain has stopped and the sun is coming out. Feel the warming rays of sunlight as you lie in the grass.

6. Imagine, now, that you are shedding the shell of the rock and slowly returning to your normal size and state. You can recall everything you experienced.

7. Count from one to five, and on the count of five open your eyes and feel alert and refreshed.

Concentration Exercise 2

Objective. Here is another concentration exercise. For this you will need an orange (or other fruit).

Technique.

1. First relax in your preferred way.

2. Reach out and take the orange in your hand. Turn it over and over, feel its texture, smell it, and observe how the scent affects you.

3. Feel yourself relaxing still further, and imagine that you are becoming smaller and smaller—tiny enough to crawl inside the orange and explore it. How does the inside of the fruit look and feel? How does it taste? Is it fresh? Does the color inside look the same as that on the outside?

4. Imagine, now, that you are leaving the interior of the orange and returning to normal size. You can remember everything you saw, felt, tasted, and experienced.

5. Count from one to five and feel yourself alert and refreshed.

Health Spa for the Mind*

Objective. This exercise will help you create a special
place in your mind—a nowhere space. It will help *focus your
attention for visualization and concentration.* This nowhere
space is your own creative space, a private spot where you
can go to relax, to work out problems, to make decisions. In
the midst of many activities, you may not have time to get
away. But you can create a mental getaway place for yourself—a living space where you can think and feel clearly,
insulated from the distractions and rhythms of the world
around you. This imaginary space can be anywhere you
want—a favorite fishing spot, a beach, the mountains, the
bottom of the sea, in this world or out of it. You can design a
room or several rooms and put things there that you might
want to use later.

Technique. Take a comfortable position. Close your eyes
and raise them slightly upward. Breathe slowly and deeply
through your nose. Now take a deep breath, and while
exhaling slowly, feel a wave of warm relaxation flow slowly
over your entire body, from your toes to your head. Follow
your preferred technique for relaxation.
  When you feel completely relaxed, visualize yourself
walking in a garden, a park, or a field. Notice the trees and
bushes along the path on which you are walking. See ahead of
you a small clearing and one very large, very old tree. Walk
closer and see the thick, strong, old arms of the tree. Hanging
from one arm is a sturdy swing. Walk up to it and sit down on
the swing.
  Slowly start swinging back and forth, back and forth. As
you swing backward take a deep breath. Let it out as you
swing forward. Swing back and forth, back and forth. With
every breath gently swing higher and higher, feeling lighter

Source: Sheila Ostrander and Lynn Schroeder, *Super Learning* (New
York: Delta/The Confucian Press, 1979), pp. 278–280.

and lighter as you do so. Take another breath as you swing higher, and notice a big, white, feathery cloud floating directly in front of you. Take another deep breath, and as you swing forward float up into the billowy, soft cloud. This cloud will carry you safely anywhere you want to go. Go high up in the air, and then begin to slowly return to Earth in a great, slow arc, until your feet are again on the ground in the spot you've chosen as your getaway place. Pause there.

At the count of three you are going to create a carpet—any size, shape, or design you like. Make sure it is properly placed on the floor. Sit down on it. You can sit on this carpet anytime you want, and immediately feel relaxed. When you sit on this carpet it will automatically bring enough energy to work on any project. Tell yourself a few times that whenever you wish to come to this place on your own, you can do so by becoming relaxed and slowly visualizing, in sequence, the colors red, orange, yellow, green, blue, indigo, and violet. When you have completed the rainbow, imagine yourself on this carpet in your getaway place—and you will be there!

When you are ready, return to your regular surroundings: Count from one to five, and feel yourself slowly returning to your usual surroundings, into a more aware self. At the count of five slowly open your eyes, take several deep breaths, stretch, and feel rested and energized.

Visualization Exercise: "I Am a Camera"*

Objective. This exercise will *improve your concentration and memory.* You will learn how to take mental photos—anywhere, anytime. For example, you can practice this exercise while in a car waiting for a traffic signal to change, or waiting in line at the grocery store.

Technique.

1. Assume a comfortable position. Go through a relaxation exercise of your choice until you feel free of tension.

Source: Sheila Ostrander and Lynn Schroeder, *Super Learning* (New York: Delta/The Confucian Press, 1979) p. 275.

2. Imagine that your head is a camera and your eyes are its lens. You are going to take several mental photos. Focus on several items in the room: a table, a picture on the wall, an ashtray, a window, a book.
3. Now select one object. Absorb as much detail about it as possible.
4. Next focus your attention on a blank spot on the wall and pretend your head is a camera projector. The mental pictures you took are now in your head. Keeping your eyes open, project onto the wall the picture of the object you selected.
5. Now shut your eyes and imagine a large, white screen in front of you. This is your mental screen.
6. Open your eyes and look at several objects again. Close your eyes and project the image of one of the objects on your mental screen.
7. Now increase the number of items you project on your mental screen.
8. Now look at a tray filled with items and take a quick mental photo of the tray with all those items. Project that mental image onto the wall, and try to recall all the items in detail.

Improving Your Self-Image

Objective. This exercise will help you *see yourself as a successful learner.* Through it you can create a self-image that encompasses all the things you would like to be.

Technique. Take a comfortable position. Close your eyes and raise them slightly upward. Breathe slowly and deeply through your nose. Now take a deep breath and, while exhaling slowly, feel a wave of warm relaxation flow slowly over your entire body, from your toes to your head. Follow your preferred technique for relaxation.

When you feel completely relaxed, visualize yourself on a beautiful beach. Feel the warmth of the sun brightly shining down on you. Walk along the beach and down to the edge of the water. Feel the warmth of the sand under your feet and how the fine sand trickles between your toes as you walk.

Walk along the edge of the water and feel the waves gently lapping up around your ankles. In the distance you can hear the seagulls calling; a little ahead of you, half buried in the sand, is a brightly colored object. Approach the object and pick it up. See that it is a beach ball—a large, round, multi-colored beach ball. Throw the ball into the air and catch it. Each time you throw the ball, it will go higher and you will feel more and more relaxed. Watch how the colors sparkle in the sun as you throw the ball. Notice how the colors spin as the ball sails through the air. Inhale deeply each time you throw the ball. Exhale as the ball descends and you catch it. Do this several times.

Take another deep breath and throw the ball one more time—high, high into the air, so high that it disappears into the clouds.

Lie down on the soft, warm sand and just relax. The more you relax the lighter your body will feel—more relaxed and lighter and lighter with every breath—lighter and lighter, until you feel light enough to float up into the sky.

To become still more relaxed, visualize a rainbow of seven colors. One by one, mentally trace each of the color bands of the rainbow: red—orange—yellow—green—blue—indigo—violet. When the rainbow is complete, you will be in your special, safe place.

Now sit on your rug, relaxed and comfortable. Think about yourself: What kind of a test-taker would you like to be?

Now imagine a funnel going from the top of your head all the way to infinity. Through that funnel, cleansing, purifying energy flows into your head. As this pure white energy flows into you—through your head and down through your body—it washes away the heaviness of the old, negative reactions, the old programing, the old fears of being a poor test-taker. Feel the energy flow into your head, down your neck, through your chest, down your arms and into your hands and fingers. Feel the energy flow through your torso and down through your legs, feet, and toes. This purifying energy cleanses the entire interior and exterior of your body, and as the negative energies are transformed into positive energy you feel your real self becoming clearer and clearer.

Feel yourself full to overflowing with this purifying energy. It is now radiating from every pore of your body. This energy can neutralize whatever type of negative sensation you may have—fear, embarrassment, worry. As if watching a movie, see this energy flow through you, cleansing you and purifying you. If any part of your body is not up to par, imagine this energy flowing into that area. Watch that area of your body change, and visualize it as being whole and well.

When you feel completely clear, notice the feelings of *freedom, joy,* and *power* as they spread over you. You can use this technique anytime you wish to clear yourself of negative feelings or worries about not doing well on a test.

Now imagine yourself going over to your desk, the desk that is in your safe place. See yourself sitting down in front of a row of small bottles and a drinking glass. These bottles symbolically contain all the things you would like to be—*self-confident, assertive, powerful, self-controlled, secure.* In the glass, mix yourself a mental cocktail of the characteristics you desire. Drink your cocktail, and as you do, feel all the characteristics you put into the glass flowing through your entire body. Feel them soaking into the skin all over your body and becoming you.

When you have finished drinking your self-improvement cocktail, stand up and go to a full-length mirror. Look at yourself, and see and feel yourself becoming the person that you would like to be. Realize that you *are* now that person. Know that you will succeed in anything you want to do on any exam you are about to take. If you lacked confidence, or felt powerless, now claim your own power and see yourself as *confident, assertive, prepared, knowledgeable.* Feel yourself becoming a totally balanced person. Let yourself become the person that you want to be, and know that you already are that person. Realize that the self-improvement cocktail you drank will continue to take effect within you, and that all the things you desire will continue to become a part of you.

When you are ready, bring yourself back to your regular world: Count from one to five. As you count, hear yourself slowly returning to your usual surroundings and into a more aware self. At the count of five, slowly open your eyes. Take several deep breaths and feel rested and energized.